Prostate Cancer

My Journey

Michael Fry

Table of Contents

Acknowledgements:

I wish to thank my partner Carolyn and those others in whom I have confided. I give special thanks to the medical professionals that I have consulted with and who have treated me over the years. The nursing staff and doctors at the Hobart Private Hospital, RHH and Calvary Hospital who are wonderful people.

Cover by Angie @ pro_ebookcovers

Forward

There is a plethora of information for men about Prostate Cancer today. This is most easily found online, and the list of advice, articles, medical reports, books and statistical data seems almost endless. For me, I found the forums containing experiences of those suffering, in particular, to be both comforting and helpful as I struggled with accepting my own condition. It is often said that, regardless of your own suffering, there is always someone is a worse situation. Whilst I derive no comfort from the suffering of others, I did find some solace in the fact that I was not alone and that I could empathise with my fellow man. I have no medical training and make no medical recommendations to anyone who has, or suspects they have, prostate cancer. I am a patient, and this is the story of my journey and I hope the following pages help in some small way.

I normally approach most issues in my life in a light-hearted and positive way. My recent published book on the hospitality industry "Your Guest is as Good as Mine" reflected both my humour and attitude to the many calamities that occur almost daily. The subject of Prostate Cancer is not a humorous one and whilst I can recall a few instances where I derived a few laughs out of a specific incident, compassion and understanding are far more important to those of us suffering from the disease. There is nothing funny about trying to urinate with a full bladder and just a few drops of urine falling into the pan. Haemorrhoids, on the other hand are painful, annoying and rarely life-threatening. They will be a more appropriate subject for a humorous tome and, as I suffer from them as well, I will be able to write with authority.

Chapter 1

I lived in a small rural town that unfortunately had a continual rotation of doctors during a ten-year period. We were then fortunate to have a very experienced, semi-retired surgeon, move to the town and set up practice. This was 2004 and I was 55 years old. Our new doctor (GP) suggested I take a PSA test, I enquired why. He explained that, at my age, I should have one and, more importantly, I should have had one a few years ago. He told me that the PSA would give an indication as to the health of my prostate gland and was a prudent action for a male of my age having not had one previously.

The test, as he explained, was the Prostate-Specific Antigen test to ascertain the level of a protein produced by normal as well as malignant cells of the prostate gland. This test would detect the amount of PSA within the blood. Around this time, 2004, it was considered routine for males of 50 years age and above to have regular PSA tests.

My new GP had in fact been the visiting surgeon who conducted an endoscopy some years back in the local hospital when I required inspection of my oesophagus and prior to that in the day surgery with an episode of bleeding haemorrhoids. It was at that time he experienced a great deal of trouble in getting the cheeks of my bottom separated to inspect my rectum and more than a little frustrated at my utterance that there was no way he was sticking his fingers inside. He then advised me that he was noting on my records that future internal rectal examinations may require some form of sedation. He did take some pleasure following the endoscopy in advising me that while I was sedated, he did examine my rectum and anal canal advising me that I had some internal haemorrhoids that would need banding at some stage.

The results of my PSA test came back a few days later and my GP called me to make an appointment. My PSA level was at 4.6. He explained that levels below 4 were considered to be normal, and those above were considered to be abnormal and warranting further examination. This would necessitate a referral to a Urologist and in his view a biopsy to ascertain if any cancer was present within my prostate. My GP said that normally he would conduct a digital examination to feel the external condition of the prostate however he observed that his previous attempt at inspecting my rectum had been noted as unsuccessful. I recall commenting that I would hate to damage his fingers with a reluctant and recalcitrant rectum.

Chapter 2

Today, in 2020 and since 2008, some organisations have presented differing views about PSA testing and the risks of population screening. Considering that my PSA level was slightly elevated I was more relieved than concerned, and thankful, that my GP had recommended the PSA test.

I am not prone to panic or elevated levels of concern until I am in complete possession of all the facts. In this regard I was more inquisitive than anxious. My GP had given me a letter of referral together with the name and phone number of a Urologist and I was to make an appointment as soon as practicable. On return to my home I immediately called and made an appointment, three weeks hence, with the referred specialist in the closest major city, a three hour drive distant.

In the weeks prior to the appointment with the specialist I made some online enquiries. In 2004 the internet and Google were not within such a cluttered and convoluted environment as today. There were a number of websites containing a variety of information. Some were technical medical sites, others more topical and a quantity of alternative medicinal websites and advertisements. This was also some years before Facebook and other social media platforms became popular. I found the online information to be informative however with conflicting opinions particularly pertaining to the subject of radical prostatectomy.

My visit to my Urologist was what could be termed as routine until he commented on the fact that my letter of referral stated I would need to be sedated for a digital examination. He assured me that the inspection need not be too distressful if I relax and he could perform the inspection with me standing and leaning forward across his examination table. I was pleased to see him wearing a rubber glove and placing some lubricant on his fingers and his manner was gentle even though I found the experience extremely uncomfortable and bordering on a violation.

He informed me that the prostate appeared to be of normal size, soft and with no irregularities. He advised that further examination by biopsy would make sure there was no cancer present to which I of course consented. He told me that he would be inserting five needles into the prostate gland which would each take samples of tissue. The procedure would be approached through the wall of the rectum and thus into the prostate gland.

I was admitted to day surgery ten days later in one of the private hospitals in the city. I had private medical insurance and most of the costs were met with some gap to pay.

The admission was without incident and I found the nursing and operating room staff to be most helpful and courteous. I had previously had endoscopies during previous years, so the experience was not foreign to me. The Urologist introduced himself before proceeding and asked how I felt to which I replied "up periscope" as the sedation started to take effect. I felt a rush and tingling sensation and my next memory was waking up in the recovery room together with others who had received the same procedure.

Chapter 3

One week later I returned to the specialist for the results of the biopsy. He informed me that one fifth of the tissue sample from one needle has returned a positive result of prostate cancer. He advised the cancer was graded with a Gleeson score of 3. I was also advised that the cancer cells were classified as T1 "well differentiated, slow growing and non-aggressive". However, he said that it was nevertheless prostate cancer and that it was imminently curable by a radical prostatectomy. He also told me that he recommended I have a full body scan to ensure there was no other detectable cancer present. I, of course, consented.

I must confess that I was a little concerned that cancer had been detected but relieved, at the same time, that the cancer was not aggressive and, given the information at hand, was quite small. The body scan went without incident and I returned a few days later to the specialist for the results. I was given the all clear from the full body scan and was advised to consider the results and discuss further treatment with my GP. I was also advised by the specialist to consider all options including alternative therapy. I appreciated his candour apart from the comment about the imminent cure of radical prostatectomy; that did phase me a little.

As I was leaving, the specialist followed me to reception where I completed my payment and medical fund requirements. It was at that time that a remark from one of his staff caused a complete meltdown by the specialist. I gathered that it was caused by one of his staff passing on information provided by a colleague to which the specialist erupted into a profane and expletive ridden tirade towards the staff member and within earshot of the total surgery. It was at that time, regardless of any future interventions, that I gave serious consideration to this man holding a knife to my private parts or associated equipment. To have a clinician with such an explosive temper present during a delicate procedure was to me an anathema. I would be speaking with my GP about another specialist.

Upon return to my hometown I made an appointment with my GP. On the day of the appointment I was running late as a client had detained me, and by the time I got to the surgery I was fifteen minutes late. This normally would not be a problem as doctors historically always run late for appointments. However, there was a new receptionist at the nursing centre with whom I was not familiar and had obviously been trained in Nazi Germany. Not only had she cancelled my appointment at the time I was not present, as I was late, she would be charging me a cancellation fee. She told me that there were no more available appointments that day and that waiting in the surgery for a space was not an option. This is a small town and, in most regards, very informal and friendly; most of us know each other however this lady was from another town close by. I replied by telling her that if the doctor had been so careless as to employ her then I would be finding myself a doctor with better recruitment skills.

One of the temporary relief doctors who had visited the town in recent years was exceptionally good in many respects. I decided that if I could track him down then I would use him even if he was some distance away. During a phone call with my sister I mentioned the incident to her, and she told me that the doctor I would prefer to see worked at the practice where she was a patient. I made an appointment to see him about a week later and advised the surgery that my records were at the town clinic where I lived so they could retrieve my records. I bumped into the local doctor in my hometown a few days later and we discussed the incident, but he just shrugged his shoulders. As I later found out I was not the only patient who had decided to go somewhere else. I believe his part-time practice had developed into full time and shedding patients was something of a benefit and clearly not a concern for him.

Chapter 4

My visit to the new GP was a refreshing experience. He was younger, energetic and with a level of patient empathy I have not experienced before. I explained why I had changed doctors and of my experience with the Urologist. There was a fair degree of nodding and acknowledgement when he then asked how I personally felt about the diagnosis of the low-grade prostate cancer. I replied with a smile that I had spoken to my body and told my body that this was totally unacceptable. He gave a slight chuckle and told me how important it was to maintain a positive attitude. He asked what I wanted to do regarding further treatment. I told him that as a fully active male in a healthy relationship that a radical prostatectomy was not a consideration. I did not have an aggressive cancer and indications were that the cancer was contained and of a very small size.

We spoke about "watchful waiting," now called "active surveillance." In the interim this would be my preferred course of action and he advised that 6 monthly PSA tests were recommended. The question then came to an alternative Urologist and he gave me a recommendation based on the style of practitioner that would most likely suit me personally. We then discussed alternative medicines. He asked me if I had heard of Ian Gawler. I replied I had not and then he wrote down the title of Ian Gawler's book *"You can Conquer Cancer".* I purchased the book, read it and still have it with me in my study to this day. I will mention more about Ian Gawler later. I asked my new GP about alternative remedies and he said that during the period of "watchful waiting" if I felt comfortable to consult with a natural therapist then he could see no problem going to a qualified person. He mentioned that diet and exercise also played a big part in fighting disease. I thanked him and he remained my GP until he unfortunately moved to a government position a few years later.

I took it upon myself to visit a Naturopath and received information on a range of foods to avoid and those which I should eat more of. The Naturopath explained the importance of maintaining a healthy PH level and the role within the body of alkaline and acidic foods. She also recommended I purchase some supplements to take on a daily basis. I had explained my condition and of the diagnosis and prognosis which she obviously took into consideration when she prescribed the supplements. I still take some of those supplements to this day and have done so since then on a daily basis. The ones I have continued to take are Selenium, Vitamin E and Vitamin D. I was also told to minimise dairy, red meat, caffeine, alcohol and of most importance sugar. If I could, I was told, eliminate sugar as much as I can including sweet food such as confectionary, soft drinks, pastries and chocolate (that

15

would be difficult, and I still struggle today). I have such a sweet tooth.

At a recent writer's meeting I met a fellow writer and author Tara Mitchell who has written an excellent book on how to kick the sugar habit. It is called "Outsmart Sugar". I have details at the end of this booklet.

Chapter 5

I returned home with my supplements and a few pages of instructions including some recipes for smoothies and other healthy options. I decided that I would get a second opinion regarding natural therapies. A friend of mine had been going to a natural therapist for many years so after a few phone calls we made contact. She advised adhering to all of the recommendations made by the first Naturopath but in addition for the first 12 months take 3 times the recommended daily dosage. At the same time emphasising attention to the maximum daily allowance if I should be taking a multi vitamin at the same time.

The first year I had smoothies for breakfast using alternative dairy such as soy, rice and almond milks. Included in the supplements were wheatgrass and vitamin C. The smoothie would wash down two thirds of the supplements in capsule form with the balance taken in the evening. This continued for one year. During this time, I visited my new Urologist.

Once again, the difference in the level of understanding, and the manner that advice was delivered were like chalk and cheese. This was also at a time that surgical removal of the prostate was becoming a norm with those presenting with any form of prostate cancer. I am not privy to the PSA and clinical results of any of the biopsies taken in that time frame in my area however I knew a neighbour who had a radical prostatectomy with my first Urologist who had no end of post-operative complications and infections. Another panicked so quickly that he opted for removal without considering the outcomes or alternatives and then had to contend with the negatives of incontinence and lack of sexual function.

Whilst the subject of removal was discussed so too were the alternatives of active surveillance, brachytherapy and radiation. The Gleeson score of 3+3=6 was explained a little more in depth. The first figure is the description of the cells that make up the largest area of the tumour and the secondary grade describes the cells in the next largest area. This gives a total which in my case was, and still is, 6. However, I considered myself to be fortunate that I had a non-aggressive cancer, but I have often wondered how many men in my situation opted for removal instead of a more cautious approach to radical surgery.

I know that some of you may be diagnosed with a higher grade or more aggressive forms of the disease and faced with the major decision of immediate radical prostatectomy, and that decision may need to be made quickly. When faced with the inevitable and in the face of the alternatives there really can only be one decision and that is to be alive. My experience is that once a decision has been made the path forward becomes clear and easier to accept and to manage. It is only when we are undecided that we become anxious and depressed.

Those of us with partners to consult with have the advantage of sharing the situation. I would think that in most cases a problem that is shared is also halved. Then the journey can be made together. Those of us that are single may need some support however difficult it may be to share the situation. Hopefully there will be other family, brothers, sisters even mature children. If not, there are support groups that your local clinic or GP can recommend. It is important to realise that you are not alone and there are people out there that you can talk with.

In my case I visited my new Urologist every 12 months where my progress was discussed and where I would also get a digital inspection. By now I was getting used to them.   On the third annual visit I told my new urologist that it was the third time he had stuck his finger up my 'bottom' and he hadn't even asked me out to dinner.

I had a PSA test just prior to each annual visit and then we would discuss the results. My PSA was increasing slightly so after 5 years from the original biopsy I had a second biopsy. The hospital procedure went well but I was pissing out a lot of blood after the procedure. However, the bleeding had decreased significantly by the time I was discharged some hours later. A week later and I was heading down to the city for my results.

During the day before the appointment for my results of the biopsy I was peeing every 2 or 3 hours and still feeling like I wanted to pee. On the drive to the city I was stopping every 30 minutes. By the time I got to a friend's house where I was staying, I was sweating, shaking and not feeling well. My specialist appointment was not until the next morning, so I asked my friend to drive me to hospital as I was feeling very unwell. By the time we got to hospital I was in a bad way and was admitted immediately and given blood and urine tests. The results showed I had a significant infection from the biopsy. This was the last biopsy I had through the anal wall. The next one was done through the perineum, the space between the anus and the scrotum.

I was put on a drip and they were pumping anti-biotics into me on a continual basis. Unknown to me my urologist was on holiday and he had a colleague stand in for his appointments and hospital visits. It wasn't until later in the week that he showed up. That's OK, doctors need to take a break like all of us. His colleague advised that I had a significant infection in my bladder and urethra and that I would be in hospital for at least a week. I was so sick I could not give a damn. I was still peeing every few hours and very sore. The headaches were the worst I have ever had, and I had to persuade the nurses to give me something with codeine instead of Paracetamol which was not ticking the boxes at all.

Chapter 6

My regular Urologist came to see me as soon as he returned and at that time I was feeling better after the infection was under control. I was still peeing every two hours day and night. He told me he could not emphasise enough how serious the infection had been, and I was fortunate that I checked into hospital as quickly as I did. Infection is not uncommon with biopsies through the anal wall. The specialist had taken 16 needle samples of my prostate which was slightly enlarged. There had been two needle samples returning a positive result. The grading was still T1 with a Gleeson score of 3+3=6. Under new grading this is now known as a Grade 1 tumour.

I can't tell you how long it took for my prostate to settle down after that second biopsy and the subsequent infection. I was not very happy as this was the first I had really felt any negative symptoms of prostate cancer, which in effect were similar to that of BPH (benign prostatic hyperplasia).

Regardless, I had an inflamed prostate that I do not believe really settled down. For the next two years I was peeing every 1-2 hours during the day and waking up at night several times. If I went to the supermarket I had to pee before I picked up the trolley and I could just get the car loaded up before I had to pee gain. I could only go to a supermarket where I was close to a toilet. Several times I had to race out of the supermarket and get to a toilet and leave the trolly sitting in the lane. I would get very little warning and consequently I was suffering from urgency and incontinence at the same time. Erectile function was being affected as well and I felt very inadequate.

It was at this stage that I started wearing a light incontinence pad in my underwear to take up the leakage and dribbles.

The next annual meeting with the urologist showed that my PSA was still creeping up and was now 9+. We then went to another test in 6 months that showed 9.6. I told him about the frequency, split stream and urgency. I was noticing that alcohol and caffeine were irritating my prostate and I was therefore restricting my intake of those drinks. He then said time for another biopsy. The digital examination was showing the prostate to be greatly enlarged but no other significant changes. My excursions out of the house needed to be orchestrated around the proximity of places to take a pee. Jumping out of the car on a country road was no problem, but in the city, navigation was more problematic. I carried some bottles and empty coffee cups in the car and more than once I was taking a pee beside the open car door in a parking lot.

The restricted flow of my urine was getting worse as were the nightly walks to the loo. I found that a couple of paracetamol or paracetamol with codeine tablets taken just before bed were helping with night-time urgency. The time had come for the next biopsy. I was more than a little nervous by now that something down there had got worse. It was either inflammation or the cancer had grown. I was prepped and apart from the procedure I was looking forward to the sedation in a weird kind of way. The rush, the prickly skin and that drifting away feeling. This time the urologist was going in through the perineum reducing the chance of infection. Recovery was quick and painless although urinary flow was still problematic.

I was back in the rooms of the urologist within the week and he had a smile on his face. He said it was most unusual. He told me my prostate was massive. So much so that he put 30 needles each taking samples and telling me that the soreness in my perineum was due to all the needles he pushed in. He said, however, that none of the needles returned positive for cancer. He endeavoured to cover all areas of the prostate but not a trace of any cancer cells. He said that whatever I was doing it appeared to be working. He asked me what I was doing, and I said well I've been taking Selenium and a few other supplements since I was originally diagnosed. He said we would be doing another PSA test in 12 months; but in the meantime he would give me a drug called DuoDart. This, he said, would help reduce the size of the prostate and should ease the urgency and frequency, which it has, however there were side effects he advised.

Chapter 7

DuoDart is two drugs combined in the same capsule. Dutasteride and Tamsulosin. Dutasteride is used for BPH and assists in reducing the size of the prostate to improve urinary flow. It does have the side effect of difficulty maintaining an erection and reduced libido among others, but relief cannot be understated. Tamsulosin is used to relax the muscles in the prostate and bladder neck improving urine flows as with BPH. It also has some side effects, and these should be discussed with your doctor.

I have been on DuoDart for a little over 2 years now and my lifestyle has improved remarkably. My urologist has since retired, and I am now seeing another nice chap. My PSA is on the rise again and we will check it 6 months from my last visit. My new Urologist tells me that this time if the PSA is still at an elevated level that we will do an MRI to see if there indeed is anything going on down there that the biopsy did not reveal. In the meantime, I continue with my supplements and endeavour to eat healthy food and avoid sugar and other sweet processed foods. I have continued my reading about the benefits of health supplements and currently I am taking a prostate support containing saw palmetto, lycopene, zinc and some other extracts. However, these are always in addition to anything prescribed by my GP or specialist. In my view traditional and modern medicine stand side by side, together.

I do not worry about my condition as it will not achieve anything. It is what it is and I am doing all that I can to minimise any negative effects. I take the advice of my specialist and GP very seriously and where possible keep up a healthy diet and exercise as often and as practically as I can. I keep myself busy with my writing, gardening and woodwork. I also appreciate the people around me and my children and grandchildren who I love to see even though one of us have to travel great distances to see the other.

I do believe in mind over matter. Whether this be just the state of mind or some form of meditation. I would certainly recommend anyone suffering from any prostate problems to read comprehensively on research and the latest medical and therapeutical treatments available. Included in these would be the writings of Ian Gawler who is an inspiration in terms of his own recovery from cancer. Ian can be found by a simple Google search and his books can be found in any bookshop with a good medical and wellbeing section.

Joining in with any self-help and discussion groups will show that you are not alone. Some of us need more one on one contact than others. Right from the start, and this is just the way I fight it in my mind, I would imagine a physical battle going on in my body where the white knight is locked in a battle with the black knight and of course in my mind the battle scenario always ends with the white knight being the victor. The white knight is the protector of my castle which is my body. The cancer is the black knight and, in my battles, always loses to the white knight. The battle always finishes as we look over the battlements and see the remains of the defeated, lying dead in the fields, being picked by vultures and crows until there is nothing left.

It doesn't matter how you fight your battles so long as you fight them. You have so many soldiers on your side. Your doctors and other health professionals, your friends and family, all those good foods, sunshine and places to exercise even if it is your lounge room. You also have that person inside of you who wants you to win.

Like many of you I have a few hurdles ahead of me. I have a PSA test in 5 months. Perhaps an MRI. I still have erectile problems, but I have good bladder control and strong urination. At 71 years of age I consider myself to be lucky. I have never been a smoker, but my military career exposed me to passive smoking and some carcinogenic materials. I will take my hurdles one at a time and I am still trying to give up chocolate.

Be positive.

Best wishes, Mike

Footnote: Update September 2020

I just got back the results from my MRI scan.

In general terms I am clear however there was a very small area that may or may not contain some low-grade cancer cells. The area is extremely small and the urologist suggested that a biopsy may not locate the exact spot and even if it did the sample may be too small to even take a biopsy.

So, where has the previously detected cancer gone? We may never know, I guess. Perhaps it was always quite small and perhaps it did shrink or even disappeared. It is known that a good immune system can work in your favour and perhaps combined with a reasonably healthy lifestyle, selenium, vitamin D and E has helped.

Let us also remember that your own state of mind and fighting those life battles within your mind can have positive effects. I consider myself fortunate that my cancer was non-aggressive.

I do, however, have an extremely large prostate. In fact, so unusually large at 2.5 time the regular size that the future prospect of a TURP is very real should my urine flow become obstructed. We will cross that bridge when we get there. Apparently only 1 in 100 have a prostate like mine so I feel very special, however it brings no advantages with that size. It is a pity that I don't have a penis to match

Further reading and help:-

You can Conquer Cancer – Ian Gawler
ISBN 9780399172632

Outsmart Sugar – Tara C. Mitchell
ISBN 9781925288070

If you need help you can contact :-

Prostate Cancer Foundation of Australia
Freecall 1800 22 00 99
www.prostate.org.au

In the USA – The Prostate Cancer
Foundation
Call 1.800.757.2873
www.pcf.org

Prostate Cancer UK
0800 074 8383
www.prostatecanceruk.org

You don't have to battle this alone.

About the Author

Mike Fry is an author and writer living in Hobart Tasmania with his partner Carolyn. In his 71 years he has had a varied life starting with the Royal Australian Navy, retail sales and marketing, airport firefighter, airline sales manager, paddlewheeler owner and skipper, guesthouse owner and 4WD tourism operator. He has written many tourism, boating and fishing articles over the years as well as writing 'The Ormiston House Book' and 'Your Guest is as Good as Mine'. His books are available on Amazon and Kindle. He is currently working on new writing projects and enjoys time with his daughters and grandchildren.

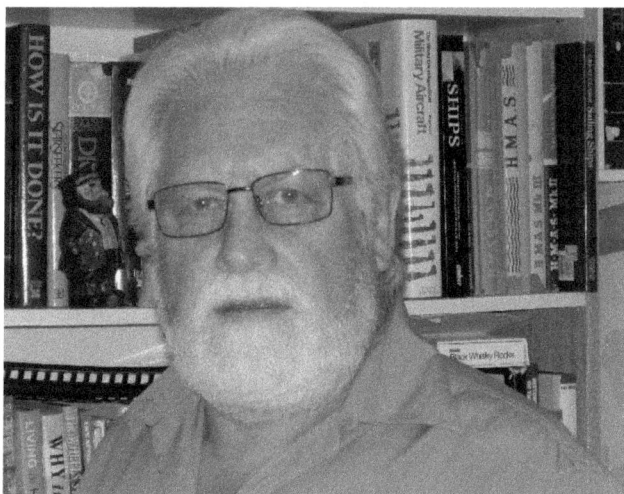

www.mikedfry.com

www.ingramcontent.com/pod-product-compliance
Lightning Source LLC
Chambersburg PA
CBHW060707280326
41933CB00012B/2336